How to train and finish your first 10k race.
By Andreas Michaelides

How to train and finish your first 10k race. Print version

ISBN NUMBER: 978-9963-277-15-5

CYPRUS LIBRARY

www.cypruslibrary.gov.cy

"There are in fact two things, science, and opinion; the former begets knowledge, the latter ignorance."

— Hippocrates

"Let food be thy medicine and medicine be thy food."

— Hippocrates

"Walking is man's best medicine. "

— Hippocrates

Table of Contents

Find more about me and my
books at my webpage
www.thirsty4health.com

About The Author.

Andreas was born in Athens, the city that gave birth to Democracy, in Greece, the country that taught to the world how to live, think, and have fun. He grew up in the beautiful island of Cyprus.

With both of his parents bibliophiles (and his father a high school teacher), Andreas grew up with a love and appreciation for literature. In addition to the books he borrowed from the school library, a stack of encyclopedias taught him about the world. A history lover from age 13, he devoured the memoirs of Winston Churchill and Charles de Gaul, and by age 17, he had read all of Julius Vern's books.

After serving his country for 26 months immediately after finishing high school, Andreas studied in Patra, Greece to become a computer engineer. With his Master of Computer Engineering and Informatics, he began working in the Informatics Department of the local university hospital, and started reading again with a vengeance.

In 2004, Andreas authored his first book, a historical novel that has not yet seen the light of publication. Leaving it unpublished made him feel like a failure, but a lot has changed since then. Eleven years later, he has successfully quit smoking and has been smoke-free for the past six years. He has also started running again and managed to lose 26 kg (57 lbs).

Andreas has run three marathons, as well as many half-marathons and other shorter races. His love for running is what renewed him and actually saved his life.

Multiple medical problems pushed Andreas to research and experiment with a plant-based diet; since 2013 he is following a whole plant based diet.

In addition to running, Andreas enjoys hiking, cycling, playing basketball, camping, photography, and going out with friends and family and having a good time.

You can follow the writer at his
webpage www.thirsty4health.com

Prologue.

One of the first signs of a person that is getting more mature is how much they help other people with their words and their deeds. People that are not mature enough don't realize that helping others is an important sign of a higher level of awareness, both for them and for the people around them.

People that help other people are less selfish, less self-centered, and they are more perceptive of the environment around them.

I used to be a selfish little man; my mind couldn't actually see beyond my nose. I was a heavy smoker for 16 years, the ultimate ego; nothing mattered the most but the next nicotine fix, provided by those round cylindrical tubes of cancer and death!

I was fortunate enough to wake up on life's little bells and alerts that we all get at some point in our life. I chose to listen to them, and by doing that, I'd like to believe that I came up on top.

I am tobacco-free for the last seven years now and going strong. That experience made me write a number of articles listed in the quit-smoking area of my blog. Also, I wrote a book entitled "16 Smoking Rationalizations"

As a result of quitting smoking, I gained a considerable weight, and another Golgotha started for me. My saga of how I managed to lose 44 pounds once and for all is depicted in my book "How I lost 44 pounds and never gained them back" (same tactic).

At the beginning of my effort, I managed to lose the pounds through the exercise that was and still is my favorite; running.

Getting older and allowing your mind to accept changes and also allow yourself to remove prejudices we all have,inone way or another, you become wiser, you become more mature, and you become less selfish.

Writing books for me now was never about the money. I have a good steady job that I enjoy, I am one of the lucky ones you can say that actually enjoy doing their job, and I'm actually getting paid to do something that I love. So, to repeat, writing books is not about money for me; it's about helping other people achieve the things I did, minus the mistakes I made.

I always write about things I know, I will never write or give advice on matters that I have no idea whatsoever like many "Gurus" do out there on the web.

I always present my sources and always have the experience to back it up. I write about smoking and how to quit smoking because I was a pitiful tobacco smoker for 16 years, from the age of 19 to 35 I was self-destroying myself.
I write about how to quit smoking because I have been tobacco-free for the last 7 years, and not just for one month or 3 months like so many quit-smoking gurus out there do. You will see them run to announce how they quit smoking only a few months after while they barely know what they are up against in the future.

I write on how to lose weight using a plant-based lifestyle because that's how I lost 44 pounds and never gained them back, and it's been 3 and a half years now that I am applying this lifestyle, and I know what I am talking about because it still works.

I write about running distances from 5km to 50km because, for the last 6 years, I've been a runner, and I also used to be a high school runner—and a very good one too.

Now, lots of you will wonder why on earth you are telling us all these, especially in a book about how to train and finish your first 10km race. Well, that's a very good question, and I never leave a question unanswered even if it's my alter ego that is asking it (smile). Well, I am saying all these first because I can (another smile)—thank goodness for independent publishing—and second because, like all big changes in your life, in order for it to become a lifestyle and for you, asaresult, to enjoy the beneficial advantages of it, you need to be informed of two simple rules first.

You need to know the theory behind it, the mindset. Second, you need to know the practical aspect of the theory, and last but not least, you need to know the step by step configuration your mind has to follow to achieve that task.

Any lack of information in either of the above situations and your rate of success diminishes, and this applies to all the tasks that people set their minds to conquer.

I am telling you all these, so you see that the information you are going to read in this book will help you train and finish your first 10km race.

Saying that, you have to understand that this book is primarily focused and addressed to people that are already running and that maybe they had a few 5k races or maybe they hadn't, but they are thinking of entering a 10k race, and their goal is just tofinish the event.

On the other hand, more experienced runners might enjoy this book too. As we become more experienced runners, we tend to assume that we know everything.It's inhuman nature to bang your head on the wall, so I personally do enjoy reading books about running but also other niches that take me back to the basics.

Here's an example that will showcase what I am saying more clearly. Last Sunday, October9,2016, I was in Bucharest Romania, running the half marathon there, and my time was 2 hours and 34 seconds, not bad for a 42-year-old that only trained for 4 weeks instead of 18 weeks, which is the time you should train in order to have a good personal record for a half-marathon race.

The funny thing is that three years ago—and that means I was also three years younger—my time in the same race was 2 hours and 7 minutes! How is that possible? —someone may ask. You are older, and yet you make a better time?Isn't that strange?

Actually, it's not, but that's a story for another book which I promise I will publish soon. Anyway, I got side tracked for a moment there. Back to what I was saying, one of the things you need to do in half-marathon races is to apply a protective gel on your nipples, and, basically, anywhere you might get some scuffing.

Guess what I forgot to do? Yep, I forgot to apply my petroleum-free gel, and at the end of the race, after everything cooled down, and especially after I took a nice hot shower, I was in pain for two days from all the irritation the scuffing gave me.

Now why did I forget? Well, maybe because I haven't run an official race for a year, or maybe I assumed I knew everything, so, yes, this book could be appreciated by more mature and experienced runners as a reminder-of-the-basics apparatus.

When I was writing "How to train and finish your 5k race," I always tried to have on my mind that I was writing this book for people that never run in their life, and I tried to present my mindset and how I changed it in order to adopt running as a lifestyle habit.

I mentioned earlier for theory, practice and an application algorithm to get things done, but also a journey always starts with a small step. The factor keys here are the decision to do something, the commitment, and perseverance.

So if you are a reader that bought this book because you want to run a 10k for the first time, that's great. I am sure if you follow what I have to say here, you'll be finishing, and you can take that to the bank.

My advice,though, is to get my 5k book also as it has a lot of information about why you should start running; information that is more addressed to your motives than the physical situation of the race.

I like not to repeat the same information in my books, but some things mentioned in the 5k book will also be mentioned here inevitably.

So, with no further ado, let's start learning how to train and finish your first 10k race.

Why run a 10k race anyway?

When I was 14 years old, my father told me a story of how when he was in high school he won a running race—I don't remember if he came first or second. If you know my father, then you will understand why I love him to bits, and, most importantly, he is the best father any kid could ask for—well, except for the fact he was a smoker, but he is not anymore; we quit together—other than that, he is just perfect, and I am not saying that because he is my father. Anyway, after my father told me that, naturally, I wanted to be like him, so when the gymnastics professor announced that there will be a two-mile qualifier race, I made sure I participated on that.

About a week after the announcement (if I remember right after 28 years!—Time sure flies by, people), all the kids that were participating got into a bus and drove from the high school onto the old road of the village, exactly 2 miles from high school.
When we got there, we got out of the bus, and our professor said we had 10 minutes for warm-up. A "warm-up," what's that? I never run in my life. Well, I did run when I was playing football with the other kids of my village, but running for 2 miles was the first time.

The other kids that knew a little bit more than Ididwere stretching and running up and down and some were running on the spot. Anyway, the whole scene was new to me, and I felt awkward.

After the ten minutes of warm-up were up, and we all had lined behind an imaginary line, the teacher blew the whistle, and off we went.

I don't remember much from that race except three things; one, I was running like the devil was after me; second, my lungs were on fire, and third, I managed to finish second which was pretty amazing considering I beat kids older than me and more trained and experienced.

Now that was a beautiful feeling, the emotional situation I was in after I finished, the joy, the excitement, and the happiness of finishing that race are something I wish all people feel at some point in their life.

Training and finishing your first 10k will give you the same emotional satisfaction I got all those years ago when I finished my first 2 miles.

So, I think one reason for someone to train and finish his first 10k is the curiosity and the excitement of a beginner intherunning.

When I started running again at the age of 35, my motive was to lose weight, and I was very motivated to go outside every day and start running like my pants were on fire.

So, I think another reason you should try and run a 10k race is to keep you motivated to go outside and run like your pants are on fire.

If you are running for a while now and have a few 5k under your belt, then I think it's imperative to go for your first 10k race for numerous reasons. First, the extra training will challenge you even more, having as a result, more improvement on your fitness status and, of course, the most important thing of all, your health will improve dramatically as well because you will lose more weight since the 10k training is a bit more demanding. Second, you will impress the opposite sex when they find out that you advanced from 5k to 10k races (wink). Third, your already boosted self-esteem and confidence will skyrocket even more, and, trust me, you will feel fantastic; you'll be feeling like everything is possible, which is as long as you commit and manage your time correctly. Fourth, you will make more friends, and finally fifth, but not least, you should run a 10k race just to see what will happen!

Do not forget to do a medical check-up

As I described in my first book "Thirsty for Health" and also on "How to train and finish your first 5k race," when I started running six and a half years ago, I did not do a medical check-up, I just started running, and the thought that I might drop dead while running never occurred to me.

Well, I was lucky; I had a lot going for me; I was a heavy smoker for 16 years, I was overweight and flirting with obesity and my heart, and generally all my systems—cardiovascular, respiratory, nervous system, muscles—were not in the best shape.

So, my advice again is to go make a medical checkup even if you had done one before you started running or training for your 5k, you should go and make one for your 10k also. I mean if you think about it, a 10k is two 5k's, one behind the other, it is a different animal than a 5k race.

I bet you'll be pleasantly surprised by the results. You have nothing to lose but everything to gain.

Setting goals

Now, my advice, like in any new attempt, is to keep your goal as simple as possible. You should avoid any complications or at least minimize complex situations or complicated scenarios as much as you can. By doing this, you have less to worry, and your stress level will not be killing your stomach or pounding on your head.

So, my advice is to make it your goal just to finish the race without worrying about race deadlines or making a personal record. After you have a few 10k races under your belt, you can worry about those things because, by then, you will have the acquired knowledge and the accumulated experience as a useful guide.

Alone or with Company

I did touch on this issue in my 5k book, and I just want to add a few new acquired knowledge gained from my personal experience during the last six months.

Now, the question still remains, "Should I run with a friend, a group of people, like a running club, or alone?"

I am still a loner. I like to train alone. It has its advantages and disadvantages, and these are the ones I want to express here in this book.

Advantages

I don't have to worry about no one. I can train whenever I want. I don't have to take into consideration any other peoples' schedule.

Disadvantages

A running partner, who ideally is at the same level as you, will help you stay motivated so if you are alone, you lose this opportunity.

A running partner will point out any mistakes you are making, either it's on your running posture, gear (t-shirts, shoes) or technique(track sessions, tempo, fartleks,etc.).
Two pairs of eyes are always much better than one, so the little tips that you get as feedback from a running friend are not available to you if you train alone.
A running buddy will challenge you to become faster. When you run alone, you are running basically against your watch and sometimes you don't give 100% of your effort because you are alone. You don't have someone to push you to go faster, someone to motivate you to become better.
That's why many runners wonder why, on the race day, they are faster than their personal record made when training alone; it's because the other runners challenged you to go faster. So, the solo-training is also missing this aspect of being challenged and motivated.

So, after reconsidering all of this information and also looking with a different eye at my own situation, I concluded that at this stage of your running, considering you already have a few 5k races under your belt, I think if you are training alone for your 10k race, you should try and find a training buddy. The advantages are more than the disadvantages, and it's a lot much much better set, both mentally and physiologically.

Personally, I still train alone, even though I would love to train with another person, but considering where I live and the kind of races I do, there is no other on the same level as me to train with, so, for the time being, I am going to continue to train alone. Maybe this changes in the future.

But if you can train with another person, please do it. You have a lot to gain, especially if the other person has a few 10k races under their belt.

Gear up

Nothing different as gear is concerned. The stuff that you are using to run now and also participate in 5k races are the same needed for 10k races too, so you are set. You don't need to buy anything new in order to go for your first 10k race. That's the beauty of running; it's maybe one of the simplest, more economic athletic activity out there.

I mean with swimming, you need to shave all the hair from your body because of the friction which slows swimmers; with cycling, you need to buy a not-too-cheap bicycle if you want to participate properly in a race and so on.If you check out all the other sports, you'll see that running is hands down the most people-friendly sport out there.

Clothes

Running once again doesn't require you to spend a huge amount of money. Ordinarily,all you will need is at-shirt, a pair of shorts, a pair of socks, and a hat to start exercising and applying the wonderful art of situating one foot in front of the other in a rhythmic or not so rhythmic pace.

In the old days, before computers and mobile phones, when people lived naturally,as we must live too and not in 6 by 8 meter concrete little apartments, they turned to Mother Nature to somehow predict the weather.

I also use some of these methods myself as I'm living in the foothills of a mountain being surrounded by birds and bees and all kind of other natural phenomena, so I put my trust on them more than the weather forecast.

Since your clothes will depend heavily on the seasonal changes and variations of where you train and also where you will race, it's a good tactic to simulate your training in the weather conditions similar to that of the place where the race will be held. I mean you will never train in a hot climate and go race in a cold climate and vice versa; it just doesn't make any sense, plus if you do that, you will not achieve the goals you set up.

Having said that, here are a few tricks our ancestors used to predict the weather.
When a storm is coming, the spiders build stronger and thicker webs to resist and hold the storm. Birds stop to tweet and go silent. I noticed that dozens of times. Here where I live, I may be out tending my plants, and all of the sudden, will stop to chirp. Then that's my cue to get the hell inside.

They also fly really low. I noticed that with two pairs of hawks that they live near my house. When the day is sunny, and there is no cloud in all four directions, those hawks are so high that they are like a dot on a piece of blue paper. When a storm is coming, they fly really low, and that's because of the air pressure; the higher you are, the stronger the pressure because of the oncoming storm.

When there is an eastern wind, a storm is usually coming, and if there is a composted smell in the air, this means the plants are releasing their vapors, and that indicates a low air pressure.

My favorite prediction indicator for good or bad weather is, of course, the clouds. If you don't have any clouds or you have cumulus clouds, then you are going to have a clear weather; a good weather when the clouds are cirrus; nimbus then it's an indicator of a bad weather.

When rain is coming, the cows tend to cluster together, and also the ones that are nursing stop producing milk.

Furthermore...

When the weather is neutral to hot, you want to wear less and loose clothing, so your body will be able to get rid of all the heat that is generated through your running effort.

When the weather is high in humidity, your best bet is to keep less and loose clothing but alsodrink lots of fluids, water, and electrolytes and slow your pace unless you want to be covered in sweat on the first mile of your run. For me, high humidity weather is my nightmare. I sweat a lot then; imagine all that humidity blocking my sweat from evaporating into the air. Yep, I am literally swimming in my own sweat from the first mile.

When the weather is cold, well, this is a no-brainer. When you are going to run in a cold weather environment, you should think about the onion. Yes, you heard me right, think of an onion. What does an onion have? Well, it has lots and lots of layers.
When you run in freezing conditions, you need to ensure that heat does not escape your body; otherwise, you will have your little tushy frozen in a matter of minutes. So, the secret is to wear multiple layers of clothing that will trap the air between them.
Trapped air is one of the best materials to achieve insulation.
The inner material that touches the skin should be polypropylene so that moisture leaves your skin.
When there is wind and rain while you train, you need to make sure your outer layer of clothing is water and wind-resistant (duh), (smile).
Experiment with your clothes, and you will figure out what best suits you. Every person is unique as I say many times in my first book, Thirsty for Health.

A few more tips about two situations you are going to encounter.

One is the so-called" running nipples." If you decide to take this 10k challenge, and I am sure you will get hooked as I was, then you are going to want to run further and faster. You mark my words, after a few 10k's, your body and the new version of you will ache to try a 15k race or even a 21k race. When you start doing that, you will inevitably run longer, and the longer you run, then chances are, you will get bloody nipples. Yes, you heard me right. This applies to both sexes, men and women.

I remember I would go take a shower after I did my first a 16k training session and, to my surprise, I noticed that both of my nipples were bleeding. The right one was worse—ok, calm down, I wasn't bleeding to death, but they sure were painful, to say the least.

Not knowing what it was, I assumed the worst, like something was wrong with me. It was after a few more 16k training races and a few more bleeding nipples that I made the connection and research edit even more, dusting off my running books, and found out that it was caused by the friction of my ill-suited t-shirt and my sweat.

There are a few preventive solutions you can apply; trust me; you do not want this on your hands, or in this case, on your chest (wink).

You can cover them with Band-Aids. I tried that, but it did not work for me after a while because of the sweat(Yes, I am a sweater). They come off, so that did not work for me.

What I found really efficient and economical is to apply Vaseline on my nipples. If you can find an organic substitute of Vaseline, that's even better because let's face it, people, Vaseline is a petroleum product, and the last thing I want is petrol on my skin.

I used Vaseline for many years; it did the work of protecting my nipples from the friction but at what cost? At the same time, my skin absorbed all those chemicals.

It was my ex-wife who opened my eyes and made me see that the petroleum-based Vaseline is not good for me. Now I use an organic, handmade ointment made out of thyme and wax, and it works like Vaseline, plus, it smells awesome.

Another product I am using, and I also saw that it helps me, is aloe gel with tea tree extract. It has the consistency of the handmade ointment I use and is also cheaper.

A third way, a bit more expensive, is to invest in a couple of special t-shirts (for women, a good running bra) that transport the sweat to the outside layer and cannot become saturated with moisture.
Last but not least, there are some new products called "nipple guards" which are super easy to put on, and they don't fell off like the Band-Aids I tried in the past. I haven't tried them myself (they're on the list of Things to Try), but I know a lot of guys that use them and are very happy with them, so it doesn't hurt to check them out. The more, the merrier I always say (wink).

Now another issue is chafing. Until now if you are not overweight, running 5k's are not giving you any chafing problems because the 5k races are too shortfor the friction to have enough time to create the painful symptoms of redness under your armpits or your genital area.

But the 10k races are a different situation as It is twice the distance of a 5k race and twice the intensity. Therefore, friction could give you chafing. So, it's important to address this issue unless you want to have the painful effects of it registered through your nervous system!

Now, you can use petroleum jelly like I used to do for my nipples, but the idea of putting something that came from petrol on my skin is not appealing to me anymore so, as I said, I use the handmade ointment and recently the aloe gel.

Feel free to experiment with a variety of products until you find what suits you best. Another product that many runners use is Bodyglide which protects from chafing and also blisters. I never used it, but I know a lot of people that they do, so I am just mentioning it as another option.

Now if you are one of the lucky ones that do not chafe, then first, I hate you (smile), and second, consideryourself lucky and keep doing whatever you are doing; it seems to work.

Now, clothing plays an important part in chafing so use your training to try various t-shirts and see which one minimizes chafing. That's why we train anyway, to test and try products, ways, and methods that will help us achieve our goals as best as possible.

With time, you will be able to effectively recognize where you chafe more and apply more anti- chafing agents there. For example, I know that anything more than 10 miles of running for me in my mid-tempo, which is 10 minutes per mile, will make me chafe severely under my armpits, so I make sure I put MUCH anti-chafing cream there. On the other hand, on my genital area, I don't chafe anymore because I lost all that weight, so my privates are not rubbing against my inner thighs anymore.

When I was overweight 6 years ago, even the smallest distance of walking gave me redness and chafing in my genital area because of the fat and the friction.

Shoes

I gave a lot of information about shoes in my 5k book, so here I am going to go really fast on the key points you should take into consideration about running shoes.

With 10k training, you will need to invest a bit more in shoes since you will at least run 30% more miles than your 5k training, so having a good pair of running shoes is important.

A lot of runners, including me, associate the success of a race with their choice of shoes, and that has a merit. If you feel your shoe as an extension of your body, then you made the right choice.

Personally, if my shoes do not give me any problems, like blisters or cuts, and they enable me to perform the best of my training provided, then I am a happy camper. There are a lot of times though that my shoes are responsible for blisters and cuts from little rocks in them, which can become quite uncomfortable while running, and that makes me lose my Zen-like state I love entering into while running because I need to stop and address the problem coming from my shoes.

What you need to understand is that you must recognize your uniqueness, I want you to stop and really think and understand that you are unique, there is no other human like you in the entire galaxy; you are a unique and amazing entity with its unique advantages and disadvantages.

That philosophy must generally be in your head and mind and particularly when shopping for shoes because you are unique and one of a kind. So, you need to take into consideration the way you run and your body type (ectomorph, mesomorph, endomorph or a combination); your weight and the way your feet is shaped because it will determine your shoe shape; also, where are you going to run? Trail, asphalt, or concrete? Similarly, what about the weather situation? Are you going to run in the desert or on snow,etc.; what kind of injuries you had before? Maybe your previous choices of shoes were responsible for these injuries or agitated them, and, of course, your personal taste and preference also matter.

18

All of the above must get into an algorithm. Then repeatedly run in your brain until you get the best optimization of it.

Ask the shoe store if you can test the shoe for a few days and then make a decision, some stores accommodate this kind of convenience in their policy.

Listen to what other people say about running shoes, but, in the end,it's you that you must choose them and, as I already said, you should use the above information to make the decision.

You are going to cover a lot of miles in these shoes so treat them like your car tires; you are installing the best possible tires in your car (budget allowed) because you understand the importance of them being of quality; so, treat your shoes accordingly.

Do not make the mistake of using your running shoes for any other reason except running. Your running shoes should only be used when you are training and while you are racing. Do not use them to walk to work or during your everyday activities.

You will wear them out faster, and you will not know when to buy new shoes. Keep a shoe diary of how many miles you ran with them, then change them every 500 miles, that's what I do. If you feel that it may be too much, then you can always do the "fold test;" if you can fold the forefoot of your shoe like a taco and get it to bend beyond 90 degrees, then the shoe is not 100% functional, and you need new shoes.

A last tip: never run a race with brand new shoes and generally is a good tactic never to use anything that you never tried in training, either is clothing, shoes, nutrition items or health products. In shoe case train with your new shoes at least two to three weeks before entering a race, you will save yourself a lot of unnecessary problems, and you enjoy your race, trust me I know from experience what I am talking about.

19

Where and when to train?

A 10 k race and generally as you get more interested in running longer races it must saturate in your mind that this is going to be a lifestyle for you from now on and any kind of lifestyles demand from you an item that many of them either really lack or don't know how to acquire it, the item I am referring is time.

10k training is going to be at least 30% more time consuming than your 5k training so where and when you should train is going to have to occupy your mind, and you should find the most cost effective as time is concern solutions.

Uniqueness is the key word here, and you are the only one that will unlock and solve your time management issues.

What I can do for you is instead of giving you advice on time management I will tell you how a typical week goes for me and maybe you understand what I am talking about.
Also, an excellent book that I found very useful and I promote it every time I get its Never say I wish I had by Wayne Kurtz. That book is constantly open on my desk, and it taught me a lot about how to find time to do my running and generally whatever else you want.

Monday to Friday from 5 a.m. until 4:30 p.m. I am at work(also counting the back-and-forth time from home to work and vice-versa).

From 4:30 p.m. until 5 p.m. I eat and unwind a little. Then, from 5 p.m. until there is still daylight, I work with my father on building my house or doing agricultural chores. My tip here is this, you should index the chores according to what can only be done during daylight and what can be done during the night and act accordingly.

Example: Helping my father pick up our cherry tomatoes can only be done during daylight; running, now, can be done at night too.

So when night comes, I drink my protein shake and some fruit, and after 30 minutes, I hit the high school track and do my training—I am training for a half-marathon these days.

I comeback, take a shower, eat, and work on my blog (thirsty4health.com) or my books or any other kind of project I am working on.

On weekends, I work on the house or do some agricultural work from 8 a.m. until the night comes, except for when I find the time and do my long run during the day, which will be a treat, but if I can't, I will do it at night, either Saturday or Sunday. If I can't train for my long run on a trail, then I will hit the high school track, and, yes, I will run circles like a hamster, but it's worth every lap!

I am closing this part with what I already mentioned, just to form it into a saying, index your chores by daylight chores and night chores; do the daylight chores exclusively during daylight—and you have an indication of how my mindset is functioning these days.

Diet and Nutrition

If your uniqueness plays an important role, it'son nutrition and diet you follow before during and after training.

I am a whole plant-based eater for the last 3 and half years now, so my diet and nutrition is much different from the people that eat animal flesh.

From my experience, being a plant-based dieter has much more advantages for you as a runner than being an omnivore (eat everything).

I am going to give you a list of doctors and also athletes that advocate a plant-basedlifestyle, and if you are interested, you can go ahead and investigate yourself. You have nothing to lose, I promise you that, and a lot to gain from researching these people.

Here are the links to my blog where you can find these people

http://thirsty4health.com/6-advocates-of-a-whole-plant-based-diet-vegan-and-vegan-friendly-lifestyle/
http://thirsty4health.com/plant-based-docs-and-dieticians/

Now, I want to address a few tips you can use as nutrition is concerned during running.

A lot of people carry water bottles with them while running even a 5k race for various reasons. They may not trust the water that is given at aid stations, or they may not want to stop while running to get water, or maybe they have electrolytes in their water, and they are trained with that, so they don't want to try any other kind of electrolyte that might give a bad stomach and slow them down in the process.

My advice is that if you want to carry water or electrolyte drinks with you, use a hydration belt in where you can have your water, electrolyte drink, and other nutrition items like gels. I found out it's the most functional of them all. The camel pack, the one that you carry on your back, is not that economical as running is concerned.

Personally, I never use any camel pack or hydration pack from 5k to a marathon. I rely on the water and electrolytes given at the aid stations.

This way you don't have to carry anything. What I do is that I always send an email to the organizers asking them what kind of nutrition is going to be available on the race day, and I make sure to train with the items they will deliver. If something doesn't sit well with me while training, then I will not use it during the race.

Example:Let's say they offer an electrolyte drink that makes me gassy and causes some stomach problems, then I'll know beforehand that I shouldn't use it, and I will make sure to have some tablets on my belt with the electrolytes that I trained and felt good with.

There is always a solution, and part of a successful race is to be able to find solutions to problems that might seem unimportant, but on the race day, they are a big deal.

Now for your 10 k race, I don't think worrying about nutrition or hydration is going to be that big of a deal, unless you decide to run in extreme conditions like too hot or too cold, which I strongly advise against.

The secret is to try different foods and tactics and see what works for you. Remember, *you are unique!*

This Book's goal

I had this part in the 5k book as well, but this book's goal is of course so much more different from the previous book. That book's goal was to make you get up from the lounge chair of yours, get your health and your life back, and boost your self-confidence and self-esteem by finishing a 5k race.

I assume you already did that and also did a few more 5k races thus far. I am also assuming that you took that first step and you made it.

I am assuming that you are not a couch potato anymore, both in your mind and in reality; I am assuming you have had all your medical checks, and the doctor has cleared you for training for a 10k race.

If you are at that level, then I have a surprise for you! You are ready to start training for your 10k race.

As I said before in this book, and also in my first book, Thirsty for Health, every person is unique. We are snowflakes in beautiful winter scenery in the middle of a frozen lake.
Having said that, I advise you to just finish your first 10k race.Let yourself experience it, do not race it, you will have plenty opportunities to race, not just 10k but longer distances like 15k, half-marathon, and even, why not, a marathon! No one knows how this will end up, but know this, you are the driver of your life, not society, not anyone else, *you* and only *you*!

So if you set your mind to doing a 10k race, then the following information is for those who just want to finish their first 10k and not race it. I want to be clear on this.

I am going to write a book on how to race a 10k in the future because I am sure lots of you will want to read that but, for the time being, let's focus on the having-fun-and-just-finishing part.

Pre-Register

As I mentioned in my 5k book, and I think it's very useful to repeat it here, it's a good idea to register for the race a few months before the event, even if a lot of races offer race day registration. You don't really want to leave it for the last minute, waiting on the line, plus paying the fee which will be more expensive. So, pre-register and have your mind at ease.

A training schedule

Like you did with the 5k race, one of the first things you must do is to sit down and write a training program that you will follow to the letter as much as you can. The important thing is for the program to be flexible because let's face it, life is life, and events that are not under our control can happen.

Just because you wrote 'I need to do something on a specific day' doesn't mean it is written in stone. So, use your head, people, and be flexible when you are designing your running program.

Keep a running Diary/log

I insist on keeping a running diary or log. If you listened to me and did this while you were training for the 5k race, then I have good news for you, you have a base that you can build on. You have a foundation which will enable you to become an even moreexperienced runner because that log will provide you with information that will help you avoid common pitfalls and mistakes you made during your 5k race, so you make sure you won't repeat them with your 10k race training.

Your 10k training log will be the foundation and the resource guide that will help you be a better runner when you decide to run a longer race like a 15k race or a half marathon.

Training Tips

Now, the rule that your weekly distance should be at least two to three times the distance of your scheduled race also applies to your 10k race training. In our case, our race is 10 km so our weekly distance should be between 20 and 30 km.

Another rule you should follow is that you should increase your weekly distance by a factor of 10%.For example, if you run 10 km the previous week, next week, you should run 10km plus

10% of 10, which is 1km, so this week, you should run 11km. It's a good rule because it gives the body time to cope with the added stress and do the necessary repairs with safety and ease.

You should have at least 2 days off from running, and those two days away will recharge your batteries and make you achieve better performance; a rest day is as important as a training day.

There are other tips, but for those who only wish to finish, those tips do not apply.

Sample 10k training program in miles – 12 weeks – For your first 10k (m is for miles)

W	M.	T.	W.	T.	F	S.	S.	M
1	Off	3m	4miles(fartlek)	2m	Off	6m	3m	18
2	Off	3m	4(3-4 x long-hill repeats)	2m	Off	8m	3m	20
3	Off	3m	4(2mile tempo run)	2m	2ms	8m	2m	21
4	Off	3m	4 (4-6 x half-mile, 5k-10k pace)	2m	2m	Off	6m	22
5	Off	4m	4(4-5 x short-hill repeats)	3m	Off	8m	4m	24
6	Off	4m	4(3 mile tempo run)	4m	4m	3m	5m	24
7	Off	4m	4(2-3 x mile, 5k-fast pace)	4m	Off	8m	4m	24
8	Off	4m	4(4-5 x quarter mile, fast pace)	4m	3m	Off	7m	22
9	Off	4m	4(3-4 x half mile, fast pace)	3m	Off	8m	2m	21
10	Off	3m	5(tempo intervals, 2 x 1.5 miles)	4m	3m	Off	5m	20
11	Off	4m	4(2-3 x mile at 5k – fast pace)	3m	Off	6m	3m	20
12	Off	3ms	4 (strides)	3m	2m	Off	10k	18

Training program source: The competitive runner's handbook by Bob Glover and Shelly-lynn Florence Glover

The days off do not have to be Monday, you can reshape this program to suit your needs. The important thing is to cover the weekly miles. Also, it doesn't matter if you do the miles in the morning, in the afternoon, or later at night.

Warm up and cooling down

I want to say a few words about these two very important parts of running. I learned it the hard way that it is very important to warm up before starting a training session and cool down after you finish.
Our muscles and tendons are like a well-oiledmachine, and you need to treat them with respect and love.

They take some time to warm up before you should start asking them to work. Warming up for the muscles is like morning coffee for some people; they need to have it to be able to function. Well, warming up exercises are like that; they prepare your body.

I always like to make the least effort and get the best results, so this is how I warm up.
It doesn't matter if I am on a track or outside on a trail, I walk for 10 to 15 minutes with a comfortable pace, not too slow but not too power walking either.

After that, I will start running for about 10 minutes with a comfortable pace again, and after that, I start butt kicker exercises for about 20 meters, and then I run. I stride for about 80 meters, and then I slow down.

On the way back, I do high knee lifts for 20 meters, stride for about 80 meters, and then slow down. I do that as many times as I feel are necessary.

After that, I start doing what I have planned for the day.

After the training session is over, my cooling down method is pretty simple. I walk for about 10 to 15 minutes until my heart rate drops back to normal.

Explanation of the training program.

If you bought and read my 5k book, you will notice that there are few important differences between these two training books.

One difference is the increase of weekly mileage which is justified if you take into consideration that you are training for two 5k races back-to-back!

The second difference is the introduction of some running terms like fartleks, hill repeats, strides, tempo intervals, tempo run, fast pace, 5k pace and 10k pace.

Don't worry. I will explain them all here. Let's start with fartlek.

Fartlek

Fartlek is a Swedish word, and no, it doesn't mean fart through your leg (smile). It's the Swedish word for speed play or playing with speed. It is a very important strength training exercise and very efficient in increasing and bettering our fitness level.

In its basic level, fartlek training is that in which you change gears while running, from lower to faster and back to lower again and then repeat.

If you watch footballers training, you should definitely witness fartlek in one of its forms where the coach has his players running around the track, and every time he whistles the players start to run as fast as they can until the coach whistles again signaling the end of the fast pace. He does this in a chaotic sequence. Thus, the players are always on alert for the next fast run.

In a more complex description, fartlek is a training session that incorporates moments of all the running training available, like hill repeats, tempo runs, speed training, intervals and so on.

Me, personally, I use fartlek while I am doing my tempo run. A tempo run is to cover a certain distance with a certain tempo from start to finish.

While I am running, I will spot a tree on the path, and I will say to myself as soon as I pass that tree I will run as fast as I can for 30 seconds. Another thing I do is when I see a small hill, I will race as fast as I can until I reach the peak. Then, I will return back to my default pace enjoying the view of the hill. You can fartlek, using time like I do with my 30-second duration or with landmarks like I do with small hills or you can combine the two. That's the beauty of fartlek training; you are in control, and you can make into an adventure, something you would do when you were a kid, or you can turn it into a very demanding workout.

Remember you are unique, and you need to experiment to find out what is best for you, what works and what doesn't.

You need to warm up and cool down before and after your fartlek training respectively, keep the warm up and cool down periods from 10 to 15 minutes easy run.

I do fartleks 5 to 6 minutes during my run. This helps improve my aerobic capacity, running economy, muscular fitness, and lactate threshold.

So, having this in mind, when the training program says 4 miles fartlek, for the duration of those 4 miles choose when and how long your fartlek training will last, you can do 30 seconds to 5 minutes fast run, or you can run faster from one landmark to another landmark or a combination of both. Again, you might say I repeat myself, however, repetition is the mother of all learning.

Tempo Training

I already mentioned what tempo training is. Tempo training is the easiest of all the training that is used in therunning.

You warm up for as long as you feel itis necessary, my warm-up period is from 15 to 30 minutes depending on the weather primarily.
After a good warm-up, you run a specific distance with a specific tempo. For example, my last tempo run was 6 miles. I decided that I was going to run 1 mile every 10 minutes, that's my medium tempo. My fast tempo is 8 minutes per mile, and my slow pace is 12 minutes per mile.

So when you see fast pace or 5k pace or 10k pace or half-marathon pace or marathon pace, that means the pace that you achieved in those distances or the desired pace you want to achieve in the future.
If you make a quick search on the internet, you will find arrays and tables with various speeds of pace and times that you need to achieve during training in order to achieve your goals on the race day. For example, if you want to finish your 10k race under 34 minutes, then your pace per mile should be 5minutes to 5 minutes and 15 seconds long and so on.

With tempo runs, otherwise mentioned as lactate threshold runs, you improve your lactate limit, which is the limit where the body starts to produce lactic acid which builds ups in your muscles making your effort more difficult, thus slowing you down.

Tempo runs make you feel and be more in tune with your body, and you can startto understand and acknowledge the different types of speed(pace) you are running.

30

Your self-esteem and self-confidenc ego up because you can maintain a steady and continued pace. Your form and your running economy also improve.

So when the running program says 3 miles tempo run, that means to warm up and then run those 3 miles at a certain pace, the pace you will set accordingto your race goal.

Now when the program says tempo intervals,thenit's exactly like tempo runs but with the difference that you will run a specific distance with specific pace, then stop and rest and then run another distance (same as before or less or more) with, again, a specific pace.

For example, the program says 5 (tempo intervals, 2 x 1.5 miles). This means you do about 5 miles tempo intervals, and in the parenthesis, it says to do 2 times 1.5 miles, which means you run 1.5 miles at a certain pace, then stop and rest for a period of time and then repeat the 1.5 miles with a specific tempo until you make 5 miles. If you do this 4 times, you'll do 6 miles tempo intervals.

Strides

Strides are short accelerations completed after an easy run. They last for about 20-30 seconds and have you gradually accelerate to about 95% of your max speed. Perform 4-6 repetitions, 2-3 times per week for best results. And have fun with them!

Hill Training

There is nothing mystical about this training exercise. Find a hill and make it your own! Everybody hates hills. I mean they do hurt, and they do take the fun out of running, but they are good for you, and you'll be glad you incorporated them into your training. Trust me, I know what I am talking about.

Hill training is the alpha and omega of running training for me anyway. When I train on hills, I improve my aerobic, anaerobic, and muscular fitness level all at the same time!

I always make sure that when I am doing my long run, I have as many steep hills in there as possible. Also, I do hill repeats 500 meters long.

Long hill repeats are hills that are about half a mile long, and the incline is not that much, about 5% to 8% grade.

Short hill repeats are done on hills that are about 200 meters long, but they are steeper 10 to 15% grade. They are good for 5k and 10k training since they improve speed.
Now a small piece of advice; if where you live you do not have hills, which is possible, and if you don't have a treadmill, which is also, again, possible, and if you don't have a gym nearby, which is also possible, then you can replace hill training with stair training. I am sure you can find some stairs to train on!

My first official 10k race

The following text passage is from my first book *Thirsty for Health* from the Running chapter where I describe my first 10k race. I am publishing it here too so you can see firsthand that keeping a running diary is helpful a lot.

October 31st, 2010: 10K in Athens, Greece

My next race was my first 10K, which I had run while training. It was on the 2,500-year mark after the battle of Marathon, where my ancestors kicked some serious Persian butts on the plains of the town of Marathon. After wehadwon the battle, a soldier named Pheidippides left Marathon to deliver the message to the city of Athens that we were victorious; he did so by running the distance between the town of Marathon and the city of Athens. When he arrived there, legend has it that he called out the word "nenikikamen," which means "we won" in Greek, and then collapsed and died of pure exhaustion from fighting all day and then running approximately 40km from the battlefield to Athens.

The town, Marathon, gave its name to the race that covers the distance between Marathon and Athens. Modern-day Athens and Marathon commemorate the run of the soldier Pheidippides in 490 B.C.E. by holding the marathon race.

I wasn't ready to run the full marathon distance of 42km.I was more focused on the 10k and half-marathon races. At that time, running a marathon was a thought that hadn't yet crossed my mind; I thought that marathons were for professional athletes, not me.

The Classical marathon is the biggest event; the athletes who are going to run the marathon take the bus early in the morning to the town of Marathon, where the race's starting point is.

The 5K and 10K races are held in Athens, with the starting point near the entrance of the Athens Stadium. It is a celebration of the sport of running. The roads that the runners run on are closed by the police, and the organization of the races is excellent in every aspect.

The 10k race was on October 31st, and daylight saving time had ended. I didn't remember that, though, and so I did not change my watch or my alarm clock, so I ended up going to the race before many other people got there. I also asked a girl why the race hadn't started yet, and she told me that it was still 8 a.m.! I said, "No, it's 9 a.m." But then it hit me that I had arrived one hour earlier because of the time difference—I could have enjoyed another nice, relaxing hour of sleep.

At the time of the 10k race, we weren't split into any groups, but at the start, the elite professional runners were at the front so that they would have a better chance of making good times and setting records.

I started running slowly, wanting to enjoy the route and see the city I had been born in, 36 years ago. I wasn't the least bit interested in making any personal record or a good time. I took it easy, and I think I accelerated during the final two kilometers.

According to my running diary, I ran the distance in 58 minutes, which is what I had been recording in my training sessions too. It was a lovely experience; it was my third official race, and I was starting to become good at running. I felt amazing. I had even forgotten why I had started running in the first place (which was to lose weight) because I had found a new goal in my life, and I was already addicted to it.

Epilogue

With this book,I hope I was able to give valuable and necessary information for someone that wants to finish his or her first 10k race. Everything I say in this book comes from my heart and is all tried and learned through personal experience and dozens of books about running.

I hope you will continue running so that you will turn into an experienced runner slowly and gradually, and that running will be transformed from a tool to achieve something into a lifestyle that you cannot live without anymore as it happened to me. And I can say to you, it's an adventure every time I put my running shoes on and go to the near forest to train.

Have a healthy and happy day!

My warmest regards,
Andreas Michaelides

Other books by Andreas Michaelides

How to train and finish your first 5k race.

You can watch other people running on the TV, playing football, basketball, or baseball. At least those guys are getting paid to run and jump and tackle. Why should you go through this torture of actually getting up from your soft chair and making yourself go through this ordeal? Why would you enter this nightmare? Why not continue your ignorant bliss of a lovely sedentary life where all you need to do is push the buttons of a remote control and then people in the box can live your desires, your fantasies, your dreams, and ultimately, your life?

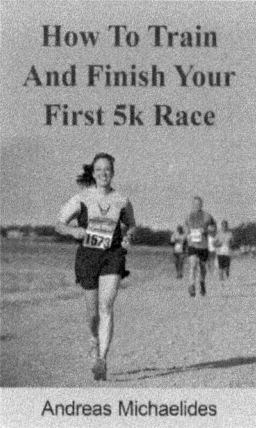

42 Tips that will make you a better runner

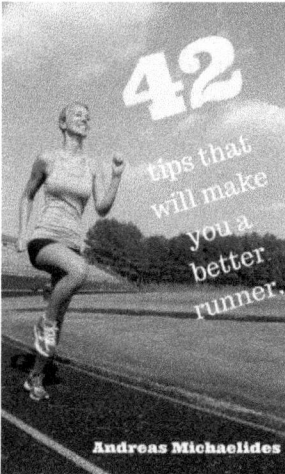

There are of course more than 42 tips that someone can utilize to become a better runner. The reason I chose 42 is entirely personal; they are not the best 42 tips or the most important; they are simply my 42 tips. These are the first 42 tips that popped into my head while I was thinking of what makes a better runner taken out of 6 years of running, from 5km to 50km, and they are also the result of a lot of running injuries and applied knowledge accumulated from other runners and books.

How to train and finish your first 5k race.

Why start running anyway?

My intentions of writing this book are honest and they come from the heart.

This book is written for the people who have never practiced the wonderful act of running on a conscious level.

My honest hope is that, with this book, I will inspire people to start running. Running is the only athletic activity that someone could truly say we were born to do (If, of course, we don't have a serious medical condition).

Running is what kept us safe from beasts in the jungle and running is what helped us find food when the vegetation of the planet became scarce and we had to start hunting animals to supplement.

Our brain, this wonderful organ, is still hardwired to tell the body to run whenever there is a need for it.

Why would anyone in their right mind want to start running anyway? I mean, running is very tiring; it actually requires a lot of physical effort, effort that will make you sweaty and often dirty because either you run on dirt roads where you get muddy or you run in a city where you will be breathing all those unhealthy fumes from the cars passing you by on the road every 2 seconds.

Also, the worst part after you finished with all the sweating and trying to avoid being killed by crazy drivers, after your body cools down, it will start aching everywhere feeling like you were hit by a truck. You will feel like your lungs are ready to explode because they cannot handle the sheer quantity of oxygen you need to overcome the physical activity you just did, or feel like someone is reaching into your chest and trying to pull your lungs out.

While your lungs are screaming for air, there is also this awful burning sensation in all of your muscles, which are full of the lactic acid that was created because of the fact that you have been out of shape for years. Your bones also will ache and creak.

Basically, you will feel miserable and in pain and all because you had this bright idea that *running is good for you*. Well, guess again. Why didn't you just stayed home on your comfortable couch, in front of your big screen TV where you can watch your favorite movies while enjoying a few tasty, salty potato chips, washing them down with a cold beer. Oh, yeah, baby, that's the life, right?

Why did you have to leave your favorite chair with the soft pillows and the inviting arms? The chair that wants to serve you and accommodate you while you can have a huge crispy slice of pizza with a double layer of yellow, creamy cheese in one hand and a nice cold soda on the other, watching other people run and sweat for you. Sounds so comfortable and cool, right?

You can watch other people running on the TV, playing football, basketball, or baseball. At least those guys are getting paid to run and jump and tackle. Why should you go through this torture of actually getting up from your soft chair and making yourself go through this ordeal? Why would you enter this nightmare? Why not continue your ignorant bliss of a lovely sedentary life where all you need to do is push the buttons of a remote control and then people in the box can live your desires, your fantasies, your dreams, and ultimately, your life?

Well, people, I'll tell you why...

If you want to read more you can find ***How to train and finish your first 5k race*** available both in kindle and paperback versions.

Please write a review.

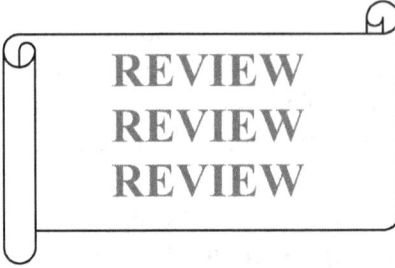

REVIEW
REVIEW
REVIEW

I consider myself as a person that wants to think that I am constantly improving my books, my work and myself. I am always trying to deliver to my readers the best quality and current information out there as my area of interest and expertise is concern which is Health, Nutrition and Exercise.

In order to accomplish that I need feedback from you and the only feedback I know that will help me achieve a relative perfection in all areas of my life is your valuable reviews so I know where I am wrong or where I have made mistakes and errors.

There is no such thing as a perfect book out there, perfection for one person is a sloppy work for other, so in order to satisfy as much as people out there my books need to be updated regularly and it doesn't matter if it is in electronic form (kindle) or paperback form.

If you found this book useful, please leave your review with all your thoughts, don't hold back, it will only take a few minutes of your time.

If you didn't like this book, please let me know by contacting me and I will give my best shot to fix the issue.

Thank you very much,

My warmest regards

Andreas Michaelides

Sources

Books

Galloway's book on running 2nd edition by Jeff Galloway
Chi Running by Danny Dreyer and Katherine Dreyer
The runner's body by Ross Tucker PhD, Jonathan Dugas PhD, and Mark Fitzgerald
Complete book of Running edited by Amby Burfoot
The runner's handbook by Bob Glover, Jack Shepherd and Shelly-lynn Florence Glover
Thrive Fitness by Brendan Brazier
Pose method of running by Nicholas Romanov PhD with John Robson
The non-runner's marathon trainer by David A. Whitsett, Forrest A. Dolgener and Tanjala Mabon Kole
The competitive runner's handbook by Bob Glover and Shelly-lynn Florence Glover
Running the Lydiard way by Arthur Lydiard with Garth Gilmour
Run less run faster by Bill Pierce, Scott Murr and Ray Moss
Run faster from the 5k to the marathon by Brad Hudson and Matt Fitzrerald
Hal Koerner's Field Guide to Ultrarunning by Hal Koerner.

www.ingramcontent.com/pod-product-compliance
Lightning Source LLC
Chambersburg PA
CBHW070846300326
41935CB00039B/1545